Let's Work It Out

A Problem-Solving Journal

Teacher's Guide

Dr. Lila Swell

Queens College

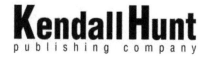

Kendall Hunt
publishing company

www.kendallhunt.com
Send all inquiries to:
4050 Westmark Drive
Dubuque, IA 52004-1840

TABLE OF CONTENTS

INTRODUCTION 1

INTRODUCTION OF THE PROGRAM .4

ARE YOU LISTENING? 5

RULES FOR GOOD LISTENING 6

FACE YOUR FEELINGS 7

PEP TALK 8

PUT YOUR FEELINGS INTO WORDS 9

PUT YOUR FEELINGS INTO WORDS --
   NEGATIVE AND POSITIVE COMMUNICATIONS 12

STEP INTO SOMEONE ELSE'S SHOES 13

   Part I -- Listening With Your Heart

   Part II -- I Hear You

   Part III -- Step Into Someone Else's Shoes

BE A MIND READER 15

WHY WE ACT THE WAY WE DO 16

LET'S PLAY DETECTIVE 17

WHAT'S MY PERSONAL STYLE OF PROBLEM SOLVING? 18

CHILL OUT 20

STAIRWAY TO SOLUTIONS -- A PROBLEM SOLVING MODEL .22

TIP OF THE ICEBERG 23

MAKE A CHOICE (EVALUATE SOLUTIONS) 24

WHAT'S BUGGING ME? Dear Problem Solver 26

LET'S MAKE A BETTER WORLD 27

WHAT I LEARNED ABOUT PROBLEM SOLVING 28

VALUE DEFINITIONS 29

VALUE AUCTION 30

DECISIONS DECISIONS 31

BAR GRAPH OF VALUES 32

VALUES AND OCCUPATIONS 33

THE PLANET YOU 34

PROBLEM SOLVING CONTRACT 35

A PROBLEM SOLVING BIBLIOGRAPHY 36

A BIBLIOGRAPHY ON VALUES 37

FOREWORD

In the world of the nineties and in the next century, the skills of problem solving may be the most important skills that educators can impart to young people.

The world that we live in is far too complicated and diverse to learn and or to know everything. Human encounters are often unpredictable and past experiences cannot, as in the past, be relied upon to create solutions for problems between individuals.

Therefore assisting youngsters to learn the skills of problem solving will help them in many ways. Acquiring information, learning how to get along with others and finding solutions to problems which are both positive and productive will in great part depend upon the individual's ability to make decisions.

"LET'S WORK IT OUT" was designed for fifth through ninth graders. It is a developmental, sequential series of exercises which incorporates all of the aspects of problem solving. This includes listening skills, identifying feelings, communication skills, sensitivity, empathy, personal values and specific steps to utilize when making a decision.

"LET'S WORK IT OUT" gives every Teacher and Guidance Counselor the activities which they have either attempted to create for themselves in the past or wished that they might have had as a resource each time they have tried to explain to students why and how it is important to make good decisions.

As you use this journal with youngsters, you will feel the sense of personal and professional satisfaction that comes when you have been able to impart a skill to a young person which you know will be beneficial for them for the rest of their lives.

Priscilla Chavez-Reilly, Director
Office of Student Guidance Services
New York City Board of Education

Joan B. Gewurz, Supervisor of Guidance
Office of Student Guidance Services
New York City Board of Education

ACKNOWLEDGMENT

I would like to express my sincere gratitude to the following people without whose support and suggestions this book would have been lesser than it is.

Marsha Lipsitz, Art Teacher in Manhattan's District 4, created and edited some of the formats for the techniques in the book, as well as illustrating the lively, fun artwork that adds so much to its excitment.

The graphic designer, Ronnie Tuft, did a splendid job of weaving disparate elements into a handsome whole.

Joan Gewurz, Supervisor of Guidance, NYC Board of Education, Office of Student Guidance Services, whose assistance and comments were invaluable.

Ann Paulson, Principal P.S. 21, District 25
Dianne Sandler, Assistant Principal P.S. 21

In District 28 in Queens, I extend my heartfelt thanks to the following people:

Lenore Stoller, Administrator of Pupil Personnel and District Administrator of Special Education
Martin Cooper, Guidance Counselor, JHS 217
Alverna Harden, Guidance Counselor, JHS 72
Judy Maquine, Guidance Counselor P.S. 40
Fred Ross, Special Education Guidance Counselor, JHS 190
Mark Stine, Special Education Guidance Counselor JHS 8
Judith Tufel, Coordinator of Pupil Personnel

Significant contributions were also made by my graduate students. They provided valuable, relevant insights on the operative aspects of the program.

My friend, Sandy Stevenson, provided invaluable help on so many fronts that it would be impossible to mention each of them.

To all of these wonderful folks -- THANK YOU VERY MUCH.

Dr. Lila Swell

INTRODUCTION

This problem solving program is designed for upper elementary, middle and junior high school students.

Two books are provided: <u>Let's Work It Out! My Problem Solving Journal</u>, to be used by the students, and <u>Let's Work It Out Teacher's Guide</u>.

The exercises in The Journal are designed to teach students communication and problem solving skills.

Many of the techniques included here were adapted from the adult version of the <u>Educating for Success</u> program (the Workbook and Theory Manual), and from <u>Self Esteem in the Classroom: Techniques for Teachers (K-12)</u>.

The exercises include small and large group discussions, cooperative learning projects, writing assignments and role playing situations. These formats require that the students interact with the material and with one another, encouraging them to be both actively and personally involved in the learning process. The <u>Teacher's Guide</u> is meant to be used flexibly i.e., as a guide. Thus, the teacher is free to supplement and/or modify the exercises with his or her own ideas.

Both the cognitive and affective domains will be tapped. In the affective domain, exercises will help students to become more aware, and thus more sensitive, to both their own and other's feelings, thoughts and behavior. They will learn how to "listen with their third ear", and to become more empathic in their relationships with others. The goals of the program are to improve self discipline, to enable participants to manage their feelings by making them aware of their feelings, to promote a sense of personal responsibility and to learn to cooperate and get along with others.

In the cognitive area, the enhancement of perceptual skills will be emphasized. Exercises will focus on the development of the student's powers of observation, analytical ability, and the critical and creative thinking processes. As a result, students will be more thoughtful, more capable of forming reasonable judgments and better able to solve problems.

The students will learn tools for better communication. Among other things, effective communication requires the right words to send messages that are empathic and non-critical. They will learn to respond sensitively to other peoples needs, whether these needs are expressed verbally or non verbally -- body language, attitude, etc. In order for an interpersonal problem to be solved, the parties must first agree that a problem exists and then, through discussion, be able to come to an amicable solution. This requires both the right words and the right attitudes.

Besides the right words and attitudes, problem solving also requires discipline -- of both the mental and behavioral sort. Behavioral limits must be set. An awareness of the consequences of behavior has to be developed -- "if I do this how does it affect the other person?". Every action generates a reaction so, students need to think before they act. They need to analyze the feelings that prompted them to act and see if alternative behavioral choices are available. Is there a better, kinder more responsible way to deal with the situation? A way that would create better results for everyone?

Expressing anger in inappropriate ways can be cruel as well as self destructive. Teaching students to understand why they are angry, to control their anger and to express it in a non destructive manner is critical to being able to solve problems and to be a healthy, functioning member of society.

Students learn that freedom of choice is a partnership. Freedom is inextricably linked with responsibility. While free to choose how to behave in response to a situation, they must be aware that all behavior has consequences, that those consequences can be predicted to some extent, and that they are responsible for their own actions, i.e., the actions that generate those consequences. The exercises will teach the students to "stop, look and listen" before acting rashly, to analyze the potential effects of an action, and to choose to act in a way that maximizes the benefits for all concerned. In other words, the students will learn to make healthy decisions. They will learn to ask themselves the questions "Is this action good or bad for me? Will I hurt or help the situation if I behave this way? What are the consequences? They will learn that they can be active, not passive; that they do not have to be at the mercy of their emotions; that they can control their own feelings; that they can, and must, make choices, and they can know, to some extent, what the consequences of the choices will be. They will learn that the world around us changes in response to our approach to it.

But, being knowledgeable about, even skillful in the employment of, all the techniques touched on above, is not enough. Students need to have constructive values -- ethics. The concepts of fairness, altruism and honesty -- to mention a few -- must be taught and understood. A society whose members are ethicless and bereft of values is doomed. Values influence choices. Without a set of values to use as guidelines, choices can be totally random, with an equal probability of having good or evil consequences. The valueless person is indifferent to the results of his or her behavior.

Violence and prejudice can no longer be tolerated in our society. Kindness must replace meanness, right must replace wrong. Antisocial actions should not be avoided because of fear of getting caught, but because they are wrong. In short, each student must develop an internal conscience; a conscience which will direct him or her to act morally and ethically according to their own values, regardless of peer pressure or outside temptation. We are our brother's keepers; we do have to cooperate and help one another instead of the narcissism that exists today and concerns only for self.

Exercises in this program will help students to discover what their values are and to learn new ones. The students will learn to honor commitments. At the end of the program they will be required to sign a contract with themselves which will delineate their own personal code of behavior.

INTRODUCTION OF THE PROGRAM

Procedures:

1. Introduce the problem solving program "Let's Work It Out" by asking the students to read the introduction in their Journal. After they have done this open the class for questions.

2. Explain the goals of the program and record them on the blackboard. Answer any questions the students may have.

3. Discuss the "Bill of Rights". Ask each member of the class to give an example of each of the "Rights".

4. Divide the class into small groups and have the students share their own examples, or stories, illustrating each of the "Rights" with one another.

5. Choose a reporter from each group who will share the group's stories with the rest of the class.

ARE YOU LISTENING?

Aim: To help students become self disciplined by teaching them good listening habits.

Statements for Discussion:

- Good listening habits are essential to problem solving because it involves listening to ourselves and others.

- Good listening is important because it helps us gain information, shows respect, and makes the speaker feel appreciated and important.

Procedures:

1. Review and discuss the "Rules for Good Listening". Write each rule on the blackboard.

2. Demonstrate "effective listening" by asking a volunteer to share a recent experience with the class and then have the class retell the story.

3. Ask the class to incorporate the rules of good listening behavior while the person is talking.

4. Divide the class into pairs. Have one student share a recent positive experience with his/her partner. Then have the listener retell the story. Then have the pair switch roles. Have the pair compose a list of the rules of good listening they employed.

5. Divide the class into groups of five and have each group do the same exercise. After the entire group has finished relating their experiences, ask each individual to "retell" what each group member said.

6. Have each student discuss his/her feelings as their story was retold by the group members. (How did it feel to be listened to? How did it feel to have each group member remember what you said?)

RULES FOR GOOD LISTENING

<u>You are Paying Attention if you are:</u>

- Looking directly at the the person speaking to you

- Not Looking bored

- Not Looking at your watch

- Not Reading a book

- Not Writing or doodling

- Sitting still

- Not Playing with stuff

- Not Raising my hand when someone is talking.

- Not Making faces

- Listening quietly

- Not Laughing

- Not Talking

FACE YOUR FEELINGS

Aim: To help students to identify, become aware of and to accept their positive and negative emotions.

Statements for Discussion:

- Feelings are positive and negative reactions to situations and events that we experience inside ourselves.

- People react to situations differently. Each person will have a unique response which will trigger a separate set of feelings.

- Awareness of feelings leads to better control and management.

- In order to communicate effectively we need to understand our own feelings. Problem solving depends on effective communication.

Procedures:

1. Refer to the "Face Your Feelings" exercise in the Journal and have the class read the "List of Feelings". As an example of this exercise, have students discuss recent positive events in which they participated and which triggered positive feelings.

2. Have the students complete the first part of the "Face Your Feelings" exercise in the Journal.

3. Discuss the different feelings engendered by the situations in the exercise. Compare the similarities and differences in the student's responses.

4. Ask the students to describes other situations that would trigger similar feelings.

5. Have the students do the second part of the exercise "Describe Your Feelings" in the Journal.

6. Have the students share the feelings and experiences that the exercise elicited.

PEP TALK

Aim: To help students understand how thoughts affect feelings and to learn how to transform negative thoughts to positive ones.

Statements for Discussion:

- Our feelings are controlled by our thoughts. Negative thoughts or "self-talk" makes us feel bad; positive "self-talk" makes us feel good. It's what we say to ourselves that causes unhappy feelings.

- Thoughts can change through self discipline and practice. We can learn to change our thinking.

- Negative thoughts about another person can influence our feelings about them.

- In order to communicate with self and others, we need to understand how our thoughts affect feelings. This makes for good problem solving.

Procedures:

1. Discuss the processes for changing "Ways to Change Your Thinking" in the "Pep Talk" exercise in the Journal.

2. Give examples of situations when negative thoughts toward another person were generated i.e., "My sister broke my tape recorder. It was a present."

Negative "Self-Talk"	Positive "Self-Talk"
I hate her. She's jealous.	It was an accident. (or, She's feeling bad because she didn't get a present.

3. Separate the class into pairs. Give each pair an example of positive and negative "self talk" from the Journal and have them role play. Discuss their reactions and the effect of both dialogues.

4. Have the students complete the bubble exercise in the Journal.

5. For homework have students use the "Ways to Change Your Thinking" list by applying the process to a situation they may encounter that engenders negative feelings. (Use this format in the "Pep Talk" exercise in the Journal.)

PUT YOUR FEELINGS INTO WORDS

Aim: To help students learn how to verbalize their feelings positively.

Statements for Discussion:

- Communication occurs when you use words or body language to let another person know how you are feeling and what you are thinking.

- The more we are able to exercise self control, the more we will be able to express our feelings in a direct, positive way. Words can cause pain. Think before speaking. The words we speak have consequences to self and others. Once spoken, words can never be recovered.

- Effective communication is a two way process. Both parties need to listen and to send clear, direct messages in a timely manner. Most of all, each party must understand his or her own feelings and thoughts, as well as the other persons feelings and thoughts.

Procedures:

1. Refer back to the previous exercises and refresh the student's memory about how to get in touch with their own thoughts and feelings. Discuss the negative and positive communication list.

2. Divide the class into small groups and ask them to come up with effective and ineffective ways to communicate thoughts and feelings, i.e., describe words and phrases that make them feel bad and those that make them feel good. Make a list of these feelings.

3. Choose a recorder in each group who will communicate the group's list to the class.

4. Explain what "I Messages" and "You Messages" mean. A "you message" is blaming and accusatory. An "I message" is a direct expression of your feelings and thoughts. i.e., A person is late for an appointment:
    <u>"You message"</u>: "You are unreliable."
    <u>"I message"</u>: I feel upset and angry that you kept me waiting.

5. Complete the "You and I Bubble" exercise in the Journal. (Discuss the student's responses and compare with the "You and I" statement sheet.)

6. Divide the class into pairs. Have each pair role play the "You and I" statement they wrote in the bubble. Have other students describe to the class the feelings they experienced when they were enacting the "You and I" messages.

7. Have students create new situations and give "You and I" statements. Have the class role play these new situations. Finally, have a class discussion about their reactions.

PUT YOUR FEELINGS INTO WORDS

NEGATIVE AND POSITIVE COMMUNICATIONS

The following is a list of negative and positive ways to communicate your feelings and emotions to others:

Negative Communications:

- Negative criticism: "You did that all wrong."

- Using nasty, mean words and phrases: "You're stupid." "You're a wimp."

- Being judgmental: "You're bad for feeling angry."

- Denial: "I don't feel anything."

- Blaming others: "It's all your fault. I didn't do anything wrong."

- Blaming yourself: "It's totally my fault. I was completely wrong."

Positive Communication:

1. Sending "I" messages. Explaining how you feel without blaming the other person: "I feel upset and angry that you kept me waiting for over an hour."

2. Giving constructive, well rounded, criticism. Emphasizing the positives along with the negatives: "Gee you worked so hard on that project, what a shame it didn't turn out better. I think maybe you were pressed for time. What about starting a little earlier next time?"

3. Be aware and respect your and other people's feelings.

4. Review the "You and I Messages" in the Journal to further see the difference between negative and positive communication.

STEP INTO SOMEONE ELSE'S SHOES

Aim: To help students to become more perceptive, sensitive and empathic toward the feelings of others.

Statements for Discussion:

- Empathy is the ability to understand another person's feelings, thoughts and behavior.

- Empathy is necessary for communication and problem solving. There are two or more people involved with different feelings, etc. Problem solving and communication can't be effective unless there is an understanding of both person's feeling, attitudes, etc.

- Walk in the other person's shoes and see what their perception is from his/her point of view.

- Responses, both verbally and behaviorally, to another person's behavior depend on understanding, i.e., what you say to another person depends on your understanding of their feelings.

Procedures:

1. Refer to the "Step Into Someone Else's Shoes" exercise in the journal (Part I "Listening With Your Heart"). Ask the class to read all the sentences in the exercise. When each sentence has been read, ask the students to close their eyes and imagine themselves in the other person's place, i.e., what is the person thinking, feeling, doing? Discuss each sentence with the class.

2. Select one or more of the situations in the exercise and ask for student volunteers to role play. Then have the volunteers reverse roles and replay the situation. This will allow the students to know how it feels from both points of view.

3. Have the students complete the "Step Into Someone Else's Shoes" exercise (Part I "Listening With Your Heart") in the Journal.

4. Review the concepts of responsive listening and then have the students complete Parts II and III of the "Step Into Someone Else's Shoes" exercise in the Journal. ("I Hear You and "Step Into Someone Else's Shoes")

5. Select a book from the bibliography and have the students write a composition on the character's feelings and thoughts -- to step into his/her shoes.

BE A MIND READER

Aim: To help students understand the underlying feelings and thoughts behind verbal statements and to use this knowledge in their verbal responses to one another.

Statements for Discussion:

- What people say and what they are thinking may be quite different. What one says, might not reflect one's true feelings.

- Understanding of underlying feelings and thoughts behind overt statements are necessary for problem solving. We need to reach beyond the spoken words.

- Actions speak louder than words. i.e., a person says "trust me" and then proceeds to cheat you in a deal you made together.

- Look at non-verbal behavior. Are there contradictions between the words spoken and non-verbal gestures. i.e., a person says "I love you" but his hand is clenched into a fist.

- Verbal responses should reflect the feelings and thoughts of the other person.

Procedures:

1. Have students do the "Be a Mind Reader" exercise in the Journal. Discuss the example before students do the exercise.

2. After the students complete the exercise, discuss their response statements with the entire class.

3. Divide the class into pairs. Have each pair role play "responsive statements" with one another.

4. Discuss the student's reactions to the statements.

5. For homework, have the students try to guess what someone else is thinking and feeling before responding to their overt statements.

WHY WE ACT THE WAY WE DO

Aim: To help students understand the motivations underlying behavior.

Statement for Discussion:

- People's behavior is purposeful They behave in certain ways because of reasons (motivations).

- In order to solve problems we need to look for the underlying reasons for their actions and/or behavior.

Procedures:

1. Have students discuss the motivation list -- the "Why We Act the Way We Do" exercise in the Journal. (Make sure that the students understand the list.)

2. Have students complete the "Why We Act the Way We Do" exercise in the Journal.

3. Have students read a book from the bibliography in the back of the Journal.

4. Have students write a composition describing the underlying motivations for the character's behavior in the book. (Use the motivation list as a guide: i.e., power, recognition, approval, self-esteem, vengeance.)

5. Choose several compositions and discuss with the class the motivations of the characters in the book the students read.

LET'S PLAY DETECTIVE

Aim: To help students understand that behavior has underlying causes and to deepen their analytical thinking and imagination.

Procedures:

1. Review concepts and exercises in the previous two exercises.

2. Tell the class that you are going to approach this lesson in the opposite way -- i.e., we will be looking at behavior first and then play detective and guess the reasons for the behavior. (In the previous exercise, they were asked to look at the reasons and then predict the behavior.)

3. Have students complete the "Let's Play Detective" exercise in the Journal.

WHAT'S MY PERSONAL STYLE OF PROBLEM SOLVING?

Aim: To help students understand various styles of problem solving.

Statements for Discussion:

- The successful resolution of a problem is dependent on the style used. Certain styles, aggressive and submissive for example, are not conducive to problem solving.

- The most constructive mode, or style, is <u>Compromise</u>. Each person has to give up something so that both parties needs are met, at least partially. Compromise involves <u>assertion</u> of one's own needs and feelings without hostility.

Procedures:

1. Review concepts of self awareness and communication in the previous exercises.

    - Understanding feelings of self and others
    - Understanding thoughts of self and others
    - Understanding motivations, reasons for behavior, of self and others
    - Positive communication of thoughts and feelings within self and others

    The above understanding and skills are necessary in order for students to begin to problem solve.

2. Explain and define the various styles of problem solving. Give an example of each style -- aggressive, submissive and compromise. For example:

    - Aggressive mode -- Blaming, hostile words or behavior
    - Submissive mode -- giving in, acting like a victim
    - Compromise -- I give a little; you give a little, trading, sharing

3. Have students give examples of each style.

4. Have students complete the "What's My Style" exercise in the Journal.

5. Discuss the answers with the entire class.

6. For homework, have the students read one of the the books on conflict from the bibliography in the Teacher's Guide.

7. Have the students write a composition on the various styles used by the characters in the book to solve their problems.

CHILL OUT

Aim: To help students learn self discipline in controlling their anger and to modify their aggressive style and responses to interpersonal problems.

Statements for Discussion:

- "Think before you act." Acting out anger immediately can get us into trouble.

- Anger is provoked by different sets of circumstances and events and people respond and react to situations differently (i.e., what makes one person angry may not make another person angry.)

- There are appropriate and inappropriate ways to express anger. What we do and say has an effect on others. Our actions have consequences.

- Using violence, verbal and physical abuse, the aggressive style, are the least effective ways to deal with problems. All parties are hurt. Anger can get us into trouble. Assertion is different from aggression Assertion is not hostile or abusive.

Procedures:

1. Have the students discuss negative ways to deal with anger. Discuss with the class a hypothetical situation that started when one person said something mean about another, e.g., made a racial slur. How did people in history deal with prejudice and hostile comments.

2. Write the student's ideas on the blackboard.

3. Have the students discuss positive ways of dealing with anger that are illustrated in the "Chill Out" exercise in the Journal.

4. Ask students to describe situations and/or people's behavior that made them angry. Record this "anger list" on the board. Discuss the reasons for the anger.

5. See if there are common events/behaviors that make all students angry.

6. Ask for volunteers to role play the "Anger List". Students should use the positive and negative responses that are illustrated in the Journal.

7. Divide the class into pairs. Have one person of the pair act out the negative responses and the other person act out the positives.

8. Complete the "Chill Out" exercise in the Journal.

9. Each week have a gripe session to help students ventilate and practice verbalizing their anger in appropriate ways.

STAIRWAY TO SOLUTIONS

A PROBLEM SOLVING MODEL

Aim: To teach students how to solve problems using the steps embodied in the problem solving model. (Stairway to Solutions)

Statement for Discussion:

- Problem solving is a structured process involving many steps.

Procedures:
1. Record the "Problem Solving Model" On the blackboard.

   a. Define the Problem -- put the problem into words.

   b. Identify tentative solutions -- brainstorm for possible solutions.

   c. Examine the proposed solutions and determine the effect of each solution on the people involved.

   d. Select a solution.

   e. Evaluate the outcome.

   f. Break the solution down into steps -- identify the actions that each participant will have to take to solve the problem.

2. Have the students discuss examples of a problem which illustrates the five step model.

3. Have the students do the exercise on the five problem steps.

4. Discuss the overview of the "Problem Solving Model". Each of the five steps in the model will be treated separately in the following exercises in the Journal and in the Teacher's Guide.

TIP OF THE ICEBERG

Aim: To help students understand how to define a problem.

Statements for Discussion:

- The problem as presented is not always the real or underlying problem.

- An interpersonal problem is a conflict between two or more persons. (Personal problems are internal conflicts with yourself.)

- Problems can't be solved unless the problem is defined.

- Choose your battles -- not all problems are worth fighting for.

Procedures:

1. Ask student volunteers to present an interpersonal problem to the class. Record each problem on the blackboard.

2. Divide the class into small groups and have each group define several problems that were listed on the blackboard. Have one member of each group act as the recording secretary and write down the problem definitions suggested by the group members.

3. Have the groups reduce each of the problems to a Book Title or a Newspaper Headline.

4. Have the group speculate about what may lay beneath the problem as stated. Is there more than meets the eye? What shows and what doesn't show?

5. Have the groups submit their definitions and have the class collaborate and come up with a unanimous definition of the problem.

6. Have the students complete "The Tip of The Iceberg" exercise in the Journal.

MAKE A CHOICE (EVALUATE SOLUTIONS)

Aim: To teach students to think through solutions to problems and to recognize that each solution has a consequence.

Statements for Discussion:

- There are both self defeating (negative) and self fulfilling (positive) choices.

    a. A self defeating choice is one that hurts or is bad for us.

    b. A self fulfilling choice is one that helps us to grow, is healthy and is good for us.

- In order to choose the best solution(s) to problems, the consequences of the actions and behavior required by each particular solution need to be thought through. For instance, one must ask oneself the questions "if I choose to solve the problem in this way, what will happen? How will the other person respond? What do I want the end result to be? What are my goals?"

Procedures:

1. Choose several problem solving letters from the "Dear Problem Solver" exercise in the Journal.

2. Brainstorm all possible solutions in small groups (all solutions are valid except anti social ones)

3. Choose a reporter from each of the small groups and have them each present their findings to the entire class.

4. The entire class then selects a solution after examining the outcomes and consequences of each choice.

5. Have the class do the "Make a Choice" exercise in the Journal.

6. Discuss each choice, one at a time. Ask the students to explain what the consequences of each choice are.

7. Have students role play the situations in the "Make a Choice" exercise. Then have the students decide which response would be the most effective way to deal with this problem.

8. Tell a story in which characters are in conflict. (Alternatively, have the class read a story from one of the books in the bibliography in the back of the Teacher's Guide.) Stop before there is a resolution of the conflict. Have the students describe and evaluate the solutions. Now read the end of the story and have the students determine whether they agree with the conclusion.

WHAT'S BUGGING ME?

Aim: To help students apply the problem solving model to their own problems.

Procedures:

1. Review the problem solving model.

   a. Define the problem.
   b. Generate solutions.
   c. Evaluate solutions.
   d. Select a solution.
   e. Evaluate the outcome.

2. Have the class members write an anonymous problem on a piece of paper and put it into the "problem box".

3. Divide the class into groups of five. Have each group select a problem from the box and then have the group solve the problem using the "What's Bugging Me" letter.

4. Have students select a problem they have and complete the "What's Bugging Me" exercise in the Journal.

5. If students choose to, they can share their problems with the class.

6. Have the students complete the "Dear Problem Solver" exercise in the Journal.

7. Have the students elect an advisory board to assist students when they have problems in class. This advisory board can deal with problems through discussions or via a written response. (Make sure it is under teacher supervision.)

LET'S MAKE A BETTER WORLD

Aim: To help students apply the problem solving model to their own community and to the world.

Statement for Discussion:

What the mind cannot conceive it cannot achieve.

Procedures:

1. Have students close their eyes and visualize how they want the world to be.

2. Discuss with the class the various problems that exist in our society (in our community, city, country and world) that interfere with this positive vision of the world.

3. Record the student's responses on the blackboard.

4. Divide the class into groups of five and have each group brainstorm solutions to the problems that they identified.

5. Each group will select a person to record the results of its deliberations. This person will report the group's findings and recommendations to the entire class.

6. Have students complete the "Make a Better World" exercise in the Journal.

7. For homework, have the students interview people in their community and ask them what problems they see facing their community and how would they solve them. Have the students write a report on their findings and share these reports with the class.

8. As an additional homework assignment, have the students write and essay on three domestic problems that the President of the U.S.A. faced in in past year. Tell how the problems were solved, if they were, or how they could be solved, if they weren't.

9. Essays can be read to the class and the class can agree, disagree or come up with new solutions.

WHAT I LEARNED ABOUT PROBLEM SOLVING

Aim: To review concepts of Problem Solving and help students to develop a sense of responsibility for their actions and to honor their commitments.

Procedures:

1. Review with the students what they learned about Problem Solving.

2. Have students fill in the "What I Learned About Problem Solving" exercise in the Journal.

3. Divide the class into groups of five and have each quintet make a group "what wheel" of all the things they learned. Write these things between the spokes of the wheel.

4. Have all groups share their "what wheels" with each other.

5. Hang up all the "what wheels" on the wall. Analyze the group of charts and look for commonalities among the things the students learned about problem solving.

6. Have students reread the "Bill of Rights" and the "Classroom Contract" in the Journal and, if they agree, have them sign the contract.

VALUE DEFINITIONS

Aim: To help students understand the origin and definition of values.

Statements for Discussion:

- Values are formed by people, cultures, society and personal experiences.

- Individuals have different values.

Procedures:

1. Define and discuss the meaning of the value words on the "Value Wheel" in the Journal. Hove students give examples of each value in the value definition list.

2. Divide the class into small groups and have each group read an autobiography of a U.S. president.

3. Have each group make a list of the president's values describing their origin. Have the groups give evidence to support the values they selected.

4. Have the class as a whole discuss the group findings. Compare and contrast the values of each president.

VALUE AUCTION

Aim: To help students identify their own values.

Statement for Discussion:

- Our true values emerge when we are forced to make decisions or to choose between two or more alternatives or courses of action.

Procedures:

1. Explain and discuss the purpose of and the procedures for conducting an auction.

2. Divide the class into groups of five. Allot an imaginary $2,000 to each member of the group to use during the auction. Choose an auctioneer in each group. The auctioneer is allowed to bid during the auction.

3. Prior to the auction have the students read the list of items to be auctioned and budget the amount they will bid on each item (anywhere from $0 to $2,000). Have each student record the amount of their budget for the item in the "Auction" exercise in the Journal. (Allow only three minutes for this procedure. The element of pressure is extremely important here to tap into a person's real values.)

4. Begin the auction. Each student may bid any amount that they have available, regardless of what they budgeted. Each person must record their highest bid for each item, even if they didn't win or if they bid nothing. Enter this amount in the bid column in the "Auction" exercise.

5. Once the auction is completed the students will identify the values associated with each item by looking at the "Auction Key" in the Journal.

6. The students will then rank their own values by listing the three items with the highest budget (money allocated before the auction) and the three items with the highest bid (money spent during the auction).

DECISIONS DECISIONS

Aim: To help students understand how each decision we make is a reflection of our values.

Statements for Discussion:

- Each choice we make is based on the importance of our values.

- We must be committed to and take action on our values in order to make a choice and stick to it.

- Our decisions should be positive (growth producing) not negative (self-destructive or antisocial).

- Self-destructive and/or antisocial actions get us into trouble.

- Sometimes differences in values can cause conflict with another person.

Procedures:

1. Have students do the "Decisions Decisions" exercise in the Journal.

2. Discuss how their values operated in the decisions they made.

3. Select a book from the bibliography and have students write a composition identifying the character's values and the decisions they make.

BAR GRAPH OF VALUES

Aim: To help students understand that we have value preferences.

Statements for Discussion:

- Certain values are more important to us than others.

- In order to set goals that are right for us, we need to prioritize our values in order of importance.

- Values can change or stay the same throughout our lives.

Procedures:

1. Discuss the results of the auction in terms of the most and least amount of money spent on the items. (Introduce the notion that some items had more importance than others.)

2. Have the students do the "Bar Graph of Values" exercise in the Journal.

3. Have the students describe how their values are reflected in their goals. For example, goal -- "I want to lose weight.", value -- Health.

VALUES AND OCCUPATIONS

Aim: To teach students that each occupation is associated with certain values.

Statements for Discussion:

- People can make self-defeating choices in their careers if their occupation is in conflict with their values.

- In order to make self fulfilling choices, our values have to be congruent with our choice of career.

Procedures:

1. Give examples to the class of the above statement, i.e., If your value is economic, choosing to be a teacher would be self destructive; a stock broker would be more self fulfilling in light of your value.

2. Have the class to the "Value and Occupation" exercise in the Journal.

PLANET YOU

Aim: To help students understand that societies can't function productively unless there are positive values.

Statement for Discussion:

- Societies must have healthy values or they disintegrate and self destruct.

Procedures:

1. Discuss the values that have broken down in our society.

2. Have the students complete the "Planet Your" exercise in the Journal.

3. Discuss why we need certain values and list them on the blackboard.

4. For homework, ask the students to study two different countries and write about the values they appear to have. Give the reasons why you think the country has the values.

PROBLEM SOLVING CONTRACT

Aim: To teach students to value and honor commitments.

Statement for Discussion:

- Breaking agreements causes interpersonal problems.

Procedures:

1. Have the students describe times in their lives when people broke agreements with them, i.e., a friend shows up two hours later than the time you both agreed upon, keeping you waiting on the street corner.

2. Discuss each item in the "Problem Solving Contract".

3. Have the students give examples of each item to make sure they understand the points in the contract.

4. Have the students sign the contract only after they agree to it.

A PROBLEM SOLVING BIBLIOGRAPHY

Madeline and the Bad Hat by Ludwig Bemelmans
>A spoiled, young boy moves next door. No one like him, so he tries to impress them by showing off and doing mean things.

The Berenstein Bears and the Slumber Party by Stan and Jan Berenstein
>Sister gets involved in a slumber party where there is no adult supervision. She learns a lesson about responsibility and truth.

Molly is a Pilgrim by Barbara Cohen
>A story of a young, Jewish girl who came to America from Europe and the problems that she faces.

A Chair for My Mother by Vera B. Williams
>What problems face a family when they get burned out of their home? How do they start all over again? Who will Help?

Frog and Toad Together by Arnold Lobel
>Five short stories about two friends who do things together, share, have fun and solve problems.

Play With Me by Marie Hall Ets
>A little girl tries to make friends with the animals by chasing after them, but they all run away.

The 18th Emergency by Betsy Bryan
>Benjie, a slight sixth grader, is bullied by another classmate. He learns not to flee from his problem, but to confront it and to assert himself.

Island of the Blue Dolphin by Scott O'Dell
>The story of an Indian girl who is abandoned on an Island. She survives by using her skills and inner strengths and masters the problems that face her.

Baby Sitter Series by Ann M. Martin
>These books are about pre-teen girls and their problems and conflicts and how they solve them.

Even If I Did Something Awful by Barbara Shook Hazen

A child makes sure her mother will love her. Then the child tells her that she was playing ball and broke the vase that her mom bought her for her birthday.

Chocolate Fever by Robert Kimmel Smith

A young boy is frightened and confused because he has a rare disease, "Chocolate Fever". In reaction to this he runs away from his problems but in the end he finds help from a friendly truck driver.

Doctor De Soto by William Steig

A mouse doctor faces a sly fox who wants his teeth fixed and more. See how the mice solve this problem and outwit the fox.

Charlotte's Web by E. B. White

Wilbur hears he is going to be fattened up and then killed. Charlotte, a spider, comes to his aid. See how together they solve Wilbur's problem.

A BIBLIOGRAPHY ON VALUES

Life of the Honeybee by Heiderose Fischer-Nagel
    Details the life of a honeybee. Shows the cycle of life and how bees survive by working together and helping one another.

Johnny Appleseed by Steven Kellogg
    This is the story of a man, John Chapman, whose love for Apple trees was so great he planted them thoughout the country. He loved the earth and all animals. He was a man who achieved what he set out to do. He became a legend in his own time.

Aesop's Fables by Ann McGovern
    A shepherd boy decided to play a trick on the townspeople, so he shouted "Wolf, Wolf" and everyone came running to save the sheep. He thought it was such a good joke that he did it again. Sometime later, when a wolf really did come, no one responded to his call. No one believed the liar even when he told the truth.

The Tale of te Mandarian Ducks by Katherine Patterson
    The story of two servants sentenced to death for releasing a drake. The drake was now near death because it had been captured and caged by the lord whom the servants worked for. One servant was guilty and the other took the blame. The servants were freed by two "messengers in the woods" who transformed themselves into two mandarin ducks, one a beautiful drake and the other his mate. The two ducks bowed as if to thank the servants and then flew off. The two servants lived happily together for many years and had several children. This story proves that trouble can be over overcome when it is shared.

The Giving Tree by Shel Silverstein
    The story of a tree, so giving and so full of love for a young boy that through the years and up to the time when the young boy became an elderly man, it gave all of itself to make him happy until there was nothing left of it but a stump. Even then the tree offered itself as a place where the man could sit and rest. This shows how rich the gift of giving can be.

<u>Rosie and Michael</u> by Judith Viorst

Through the eyes of a young girl, this book explores the friendship and honesty between herself and her two friends, Rosie and Michael. Whether good or bad, happy or sad a loyal friend is someone you can say anything to, be honest with, and get honesty and loyalty in return.

<u>The Crane Wife</u> by Sumiko Yagawa

A good farmer is rewarded for his kindness and given good fortune. He becomes greedy and soon loses everything.

<u>The Little Match Girl</u> by Hans Christian Anderson

A little girl is poor and sells matches. Her story evokes tremendous compassion in the reader.

<u>The Chosen</u> by Chaim Potok

The story of the spiritual and intellectual maturation of two boys who are friends.

CPSIA information can be obtained
at www.ICGtesting.com
Printed in the USA
BVHW011815160220
572489BV00012BA/294